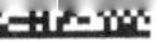

Written by Katsuzo Nishi

About Skin Disease

Preface

The French proverb says "La peau est le miroir des maladies" ("The skin is the mirror of all illnesses"), and it is no exaggeration to say that the health of the skin is the measure of the health of the whole body. In this sense, there is probably no one who has not experienced some form of skin disease during a lifetime of smoking. There is no end to the variety of skin diseases, ranging from simple rough skin and the more common skin lesions of adolescence, to urticaria, rashes, and even stubborn pruritus and psoriasis. However, Dr. Sibley clearly stated that the various drugs used by the conventional skin to treat these conditions are only effective when they directly and indirectly promote intestinal elimination.

In order to have the beautiful skin of a milking woman, it is necessary to lead a natural life and maintain healthy intestinal excretion, but even women of convenience and difficulty can achieve the same effect by one method. The purpose of this book is to clarify this fact, and as mentioned in the conclusion, it can be done by scientific fasting therapy, by following the six rules of health care, or by the simplest method, by using Klimag (abbreviation of Cream of Magnesia) on a regular basis for the elimination of defecation, and in some cases by mixing it with Oleic oil and applying it to the skin. If you mix it with Olive oil and apply it to your skin, you will always have beautiful skin. Then expensive skin cosmetics and skin diseases will be completely useless.

Katsuzo Nishi

Concerning skin diseases

Katsuzo Nishi

It is not uncommon for a system saturated with toxins absorbed from the intestines, which contain a large amount of stool, to be the cause of a number of apparently different skin diseases.

 Simply put, the diagnosis of many common skin eruptions is based on the science of stools.

Dr. Sibley's "The Tiger of Skin Disease" (Dr. Sibley: - The Tiger of Skin Disease)

(Dr. Sibley: - The Treatment of Diseases of the Skin.)

Numerous posters and newspapers have promoted high-priced soaps, pigment porridges, skin cosmetics, hair cleansing powders, hair ointments, skin tonics, hair tonics, etc. for women, claiming that these products have miraculous effects to improve their appearance. If these new things do improve one's appearance or hair, they are truly miraculous. Good looks, clean skin, and beautiful hair do not come from the outside, but from within. The pronouncements and reports that soaps, skin cosmetics, or hair tonics will miraculously improve the skin and hair are, frankly speaking, a form of deception. Those who try to look like milkmaids have no choice but to live the life of milkmaids. Like a country girl, she must get up early in the morning, catch fresh, wholesome food, eat plenty of raw vegetables, fruits and light white meat fish as a side dish, go to bed early at night, and take a laxative like Climagogue (short for "cream magnesia") to heal internal wounds so that she can have sufficient bowel movements. Most of the girls in the Yamanote and downtown areas are withholding their bowel movements. They drink a lot of sweets made of white sugar, chocolate, and ice cream, drink strong tea and coffee, stay up late, take frequent baths, and, in the best of families, dance in a dirty, stuffy room and do very little exercise. They hardly exercise, except for dancing, and their eyes become bloodshot, they have large amounts of old stools in their colons, they have lower abdomens that look as if they might be pregnant, they have what is called chronic constipation, they have headaches, and they suffer from autointoxication from beginning to end. These girls, with their pale, grayish-yellow, dirty, uneven comedones, sparring spots, bloodless and unhealthy appearance, pale lips, and dull, shaggy hair, were themselves paralyzed by the struggle of an unhealthy life. Even if such a girl had purchased the highest quality skin soaps, pigments, cosmetics, hair tonics, etc., spent a great deal of time and money at the beauty parlor, had her face steam- and electric-pressed and plastered, used artificial glitter or ultraviolet rays, and wore a mask or veil at night, she would never look like an infant girl. They may wear masks and veils at night, but they will never look like a baby girl. Even if you use ordinary soap for your skin and olive oil for your hair, five weeks of Chinese outdoor exercise, sound and rational upbringing, diet, and cultivation, such as my Tetrabasic (Western health method), will improve not only your skin and hair, but also your body. I believe that you will be able to improve not only your skin and hair, but your body as well.

Dr. John Harvey Kellogg, in his famous book, "Intestinal Hygiene, 1932 Edition (Dr. John Harvey Kellogg -Colon Hygiene, 1932)," wrote A cleaned large intestine deserves a ton of cosmetics. A cleansed large intestine does not mean one that has been placed in the colon by intestinal irritating poisons, as is often the case with conventional laxatives and health products, but one that has been cleansed by pure, clean, natural food. Mother's milk is the color that should be sealed in an infant to give it a healthy appearance. The color of a schoolgirl is markedly different from that of an infant. A girl who has intestines that function naturally and lives a natural life will have a radiant complexion. The other girl has a pale, yellowish color and dead, sickly skin that no amount of science or topical cosmetics will improve. Papules, herpes, stains, and other defects are characteristic of chronic constipation, or withholding of stool due to unnatural living, and should be regarded as a mild form of skin disease. This relatively mild form of skin rash is characterized by pale, yellowish skin with poor texture, which indicates that the skin is not in good health. Unhealthy skin is peeling skin. This skin cannot provide adequate resistance to microscopic microorganisms that cause genuine and sometimes very severe skin damage. People with healthy skin are rarely infected with many mysterious skin diseases.

As the old saying goes, "The skin is the mirror of disease" (La pean est le miroir des maladies).

The external obstacle is the skin disease. A disorder caused externally can probably be treated externally as long as the inside of the body is not disturbed. However, if a disease originates from the inside and appears on the outside of the body, it cannot be cured no matter what the name of the disease says. After all, many skin diseases and infections, like many other diseases, are not local diseases. In other words, they are not skin diseases. They are merely the external manifestations of a general state of injury caused by malnutrition, defecation stagnation, and the accompanying autointoxication. Therefore, treating many skin diseases with strong antiseptic detergents, ointments, and the like will not do the patient any good, and will only increase the damage.

Nature often expels poisons through the skin in order to eliminate internal toxins, causing rashes, rashes, small pustules, abscesses, and so on. Even if the doctor tries hard to stop this process by using strong topical medicines and succeeds in blocking the safety of the body, this may result in severe internal diseases. Many doctors do not push the disease out, they push it in. Furthermore, many so-called disinfectants, antiseptics, etc. are highly toxic. One of the most commonly administered drugs to patients with skin diseases is arsenic powder. This tends to cause arsenic cancer whether it is used internally or externally. This is discussed in my book "The Prevention of Arsenic Cancer," and even if extremely small doses are administered, this fatal disease has no harmful effects. Since arsenic, even in extremely small doses, can cause a new and terrible reaction in the body, it is safe to say that many other strong substances given to skin disease patients without any thought will have the same disastrous results. The results may not be seen until ten or twenty years later.

It takes this long period of time from the start of using arsenic-containing medicines and ointments until arsenic-induced cancer appears.

Dr. A. Bryce, in his book "Intestinal Toxaemis," published in 1920, pp. 20 and 22 (Dr. A. Bryce: Intestinal Toxaemis, 1920, p. 20 and 2), described the following

Psoriasis, flatus, rosacea, erythema lucidum, and exanthem subitum, are due to excretion from the skin. They can be eliminated by a rice diet, as suggested by Bulkley. Erythema, rosacea, purpura, and hyperpigmentation of the skin are probably due to the same cause.

It is very interesting and significant that many kinds of skin diseases do not show any progress in recovery until the patient is sufficiently treated with an alkaline hypodermic mixture, e.g., sodium dioxide, or bismuth carbonate with alkali and mercury sulfate.

This was sixteen or seven years ago, so Dr. Bryce did not know that the Cream of Magnesia (abbreviated as Kurimag, or Milk of Magnesia in the United States) had been invented in England. In modern times, it is recommended to take kurimag for various skin ailments, or mix it with olive oil in equal amounts and apply it.

Dr. A. Combe, in his book "Autointoxication," published in 1908, p. 180 (Dr. A. Combe Intestinal Auto-Intoxication, 1908, p. 180), entitled "Auto intoxicated Skin Diseases," stated the following

 Skin diseases are often caused by autointoxication, especially intestinal autointoxication.

The question of whether autointoxication, which is caused by abnormalities in digestion, metabolism (organization) and excretion, can be responsible for the development of many skin diseases is one that has been the subject of a recent skin disease conference in Berlin.

The highest authorities on modern dermatoses have resolved this issue in the affirmative. Radcliffe Crocker of London, Duncan Bulkley of New York, Jadassohn of Berlin, and Brocq of Paly have generally agreed that in skin diseases, the injury is caused by skin excretion of toxic substances, In general, they said, most skin diseases are caused by the excretion of toxic substances through the skin.

Some substances are deposited directly on the skin, others penetrate nerve endings, and still others are eliminated through the dermal membranes. Not all of the new toxic substances come from the intestines, but those that do, such as abnormal nutrient exchange (metabolism), dysfunction of the anti-glandular system, dysfunction of the excretory system of organic tissue, etc., produce toxic substances that react on the skin, causing the same disorder, the same rash, or, in a word, the same skin disease, on the skin. In other words, the same skin disease.

According to Mr. Block, his observations, based on more than 20000 analyses of various observations, reveal the following If the nutrition is too much, too little, or of a poor quality, not suited to the environment in which the individual lives, the nutrition is not digested well, especially if it is not refined well in the organism (similar combustion), or if the excretory function (kidneys, lungs) is damaged. If the marrow and organs of organic tissues are not properly refined (similar white combustion) or if the excretory functions (kidneys and lungs) are damaged, then various toxic excretions are deposited in the marrow and organs of the organic tissues, and these are manifested on the skin as various skin diseases. In other words, intestinal autointoxication is the most important factor in the formation of auto intoxicants, but it is by no means the only one.

The appearance and nature of a skin disease rarely indicate whether or not its origin is intestinal.

Dermatoses sometimes have a direct relationship to infection, but more often they do not.

Intestinal toxins are especially responsible for certain skin diseases (prurigo, strophulus, urticaria, acne, and some rashes), but it would be a great mistake to determine the cause solely by the nature of the new injury. The cause of the disease can easily be determined by the nature of the new injury alone, and this is because a definitive solution to the problem can be easily obtained only by the examination and analysis of urine.

The theories of Dr. Bryce and Dr. Combs may be considered by many to be of dubious value. This is because neither of them is a dermatologist. Therefore, one might suspect that Dr. Combs and Dr. Bryce are overly enthusiastic about their theories. We would like to reexamine a couple of well-known dermatologists. In 1913, during an important discussion of nutritional autointoxication at the Royal Society of Medicine, Dr. W. Knowsley Sibley (Royal Society of Medicine, 1913), a noted authority, stated

The majority of skin eruptions are external to a general systemic morbidity, the immediate cause of which is toxemia of the blood, the result of the absorption of morbid products from the gastrointestinal tract.

The secret to obtaining a good skin color is usually a diet adapted to the needs of each individual case. To be more precise, the diet should be adjusted to ensure effective excretion from all excretory organs, especially the intestines, so that by-products of digestion do not remain in the body for too long, or in other words, so that these by-products are not absorbed into the general system. The first sign is usually found in the color and appearance of the skin, especially on certain parts of the body. Pale or muddy skin color is often an indication of poor assimilation or absorption of large internal feces. The results of so-called liver damage can be seen very quickly in the coloration of the skin, indicating a very high degree of digestive disturbance.

A large group of skin manifestations that have long been recognized as a direct result of gastrointestinal influences have been referred to as gastric eruptions, and many other common acute and acute urticarial eruptions have been described.

Numerous other common acute and chronic conditions are also caused by a similar process. First, let us consider one of the most common diseases to which the physician is called upon to refer, namely, rash. In most new diseases, the condition of the gastrointestinal tract plays a leading role, and there is no doubt that proper attention to diet and bowel control is necessary to ensure satisfactory placement.

The term gouty is commonly used to describe a gouty eruption, but the term has a more appropriate connotation. The term gouty or gouty eruption is used to describe a variety of systemic disorders (among which are numerous skin diseases), many of which are caused by a balance between intake and excretion, or by anabolic disorders and the excretion of digestive by-products.

There is no doubt that the dryness is also the result of toxic effects originating in the gastrointestinal tract. Therefore, those who consume nitrogenous foods may often be cured of their chronic diseases if they completely change their diet from such foods to a vegetable diet. Moreover, since all forms of the disease are generally associated with overburdened bowels, the path without obstructions is the most effective way to treat them. The same can be said for purpura. In the case of diseases caused by microscopic microorganisms such as staphylococci and streptococci, and perhaps even in the case of many diseases caused by the invasion of red rods, it is clearly impossible to grow new microorganisms and kill them if the poisoning of the blood is caused by systemic poisoning from the absorption of stool or other pathological substances. In my experience, and generally speaking, the microscopic microorganisms in the skin are directly attracted by the obstructed excretory system.

With the exception of a few special effects drugs for skin diseases that are the result of the action of specific microorganisms, whether local or systemic, the main and essential function of all medical drugs for skin diseases, old or new, is to act as a gastrointestinal antidote or laxative, or something similar. If it does not work in this direction, it is not only ineffective in the majority of illnesses, it is actively injurious to the body.

Dr. Sibley's assertion that chronic constipation is the cause of many severe skin diseases may seem to some readers to be an absolute contradiction in terms. However, one must take into consideration the extremely cautious manner in which Dr. Sibley has expressed his opinions on paper. Seven years after the Royal Society debate, Dr. Sibley published his important book, "The Treatment of Diseases of the Skin," 1920, 3rd Edition, without any delay (Dr. Sibley: The Treatment of Diseases of the Skin, 1920, 3rd Edition, p. 27 and 49). Edition, p. 27 and 49), he states as follows

It is not uncommon for a system that is saturated with toxins absorbed from the fecal load of the intestines to be the cause of a multitude of apparently very different skin diseases.。

With today's knowledge, it would be difficult to name many pathological manifestations. However, it is of course possible to exclude obvious zoonotic and phytoparasitic diseases. The new manifestations are not the external manifestation of a general unhealthy condition of the local blood supply, nor are they the result of inadequate assimilation of nutritive processes or, more generally, of the excretion of waste products from the digestive metabolism.

There is chronic gastritis due to dietary errors, especially the abuse of alcoholic beverages. This not only affects the stomach, but also the liver system, and its toxic effect is catarrhal, affecting the duodenum and small intestine. In many cases, the colon is loaded with fecal deposits that remain for a long time, which are then absorbed, resulting in generalized systemic toxicosis.

Simply put, many common skin eruptions can be treated with chronic constipation. It is not uncommon to find large deposits in the colon of a patient who has a bowel movement every day. The feces you are thinking of are enough to harm a large number of people, but even in patients who are least suspected of having such feces in their system, these deposits can sometimes be found.

As the "Drugs of the World" (p. 325) shows, many, if not all, effective drugs for general skin ailments work primarily as antidotes to kill, to pass through, or to detoxify the gastrointestinal tract. I believe that their beneficial effects are not based on the specific action of the preparation, i.e., the specific action of improving or healing the skin condition, but rather on the direct local effect they exert on the gastrointestinal tract. The most common remedy used by the dermatologists of the school was arsenic, which was used for many more or less chronic forms of skin conditions. Arsenicals are, in the opinion of chemists, one of the most potent disinfectants, and their so-called characteristic action is no doubt based on their performance and stinging effect on the intestinal mucosa, and thus also on their hypoallergenic effect. Mercury is a specific remedy for skin diseases other than those caused by poisons, but it is essentially the most potent bactericide.

Hydralgol solution and perchloric solution, though extremely rare, are bactericidal and act as powerful intestinal cleaners.

I have broken every major medical work published on skin diseases in England, the U.S., Germany, and other countries. Some of them are in volumes of a thousand or more volumes, some are encyclopedias of several pages, and some are pamphlet-type lectures by physicians ranging from two or three hundred to five or six hundred pages. The theory of skin diseases in these works is the same one that is commonly explored by medical scholars. The dermatoses are specific and purely localized disorders that are caused by specific microscopic microorganisms and other causes that share special characteristics and have special and unique consequences. Unfortunately, in many of these medical books, the most important cause, the side-effect theory, is either neglected or completely ignored. Many authors have told us that each new specific disease must be treated with a specific toxicant, either internally or externally, but there are exceptions to this general rule. For example, see Dr. Milton B. Hartzell's famous book, "Diseases of the Skin; Their Pathology and Treatment," 2nd Edition, 1919, p. 26 and 38. Edition, 1919, p. 26 and 38.

Diseases of the skin are the direct or indirect result of a considerable number of qualitative and visceral diseases.

The close relationship between gastrointestinal and skin diseases has long been recognized. However, we still do not have a proper knowledge of the exact nature of this relationship, which in most cases is unquestionably complex. Urticaria, some forms of eruptions, and pruritus accompany and are more or less prominently affected by gastric and intestinal disorders.

Local and oral medical agents have been used to treat many, perhaps most, of these diseases, and they are effective. Laxatives and laxatives are the most effective remedies for many diseases, and are effective for warm rashes and other cases. Saline laxatives are most conveniently administered in some of the many aqueous forms available on the market, such as cream of magnesia and the rare Climagogue (Milk of Magnesia). A small amount of mercury chloride applied to the lower part of the skin often has the greatest effect in urticaria, especially in small children.

Dr. Hartzell's theory is in agreement with that of Dr. Sibley.

One of the most famous compendiums on skin diseases is "A Treatise on Skin Diseases" by Dr. Henry Andrew Stellwago. We find the following in Dr. Henry W. Stelwagon: A Treatise on Diseases of the Skin, 1934 12th Edition, p. 76 and 1094 (pp. 79 and 1094).

The most frequent condition, whether acetic or predisposing, is dyspepsia. This may be due to reflex action, to some form of metabolism (organization), to a direct effect of the resulting nutritional disturbance, or perhaps to autotoxemia resulting from the development of more enzymes or elements. This is where Pick, Hallopesu, and others have come into direct contact. I am convinced that this last one is one of the most important causes, perhaps the only cause, of erythema multiforme, measles, and many similar diseases. These diseases occur spontaneously in products that have undergone putrefaction or other changes prior to or following digestion. Constipation is the most important factor in the production of new products.

Laxatives are used in skin diseases to a greater extent than they are used merely occasionally. The maintenance of free bowel function, especially in inflammatory diseases, must be emphasized as it removes toxic products and generally improves digestion.

[Erythema multiforme is not rare, accounting for 5 to 1% of all skin diseases. The cause of erythema multiforme is still unclear, but from my own experience, I would like to respect the belief that the intestinal elements and possibly other sources of music are often the most important factors.

It is difficult to describe the geometric effect of placement on the course of a disease. However, it is my own observation that there is no effect, as many people claim. It is certain that the development of the intestines plays an important role in many new diseases. Therefore, the most commonly used and, in my experience, most effective treatment is to administer close to full doses of Salicyl, Zarol, or Temor benzoate. The first dose should be given in combination with one or more of these medicines.

[Psoriasis] The leumatic and gouty tendencies of psoriasis are often of pathogenic (causative) importance (Bourdillon, Gerhardt, Bulkley, Shoemaker, Corlett, Liveing, and others). Mr. Corlett, Mr. Liveing, and others). When it is pronounced, it suggests that the most effective placement is in this pathological aspect. In some severe cases, especially those developing sexually transmitted dermatitis, and in oyster-shell psoriasis, arthritic symptoms, especially those of malformant fasciitis, may accompany the disease. Insufficient renal excretion may also be a factor in those who are morbidly predisposed. Digestive and nutritional disorders of all kinds are definitely reoccurring and probable causative influences.

[Digestive insufficiency, indigestion, and constipation are to be given high priority when discussing the causes of erythroderma. In fact, in my experience, this is of primary importance. This condition can cause flare-ups in those who are prone to eruptions, but as soon as they are relatively completely digested, they quickly rebel and are cured. This is not only a serious pathogenic (causative) factor in the case of adults, but also has an even more serious effect in the case of infantile and childhood rashes.

If we accept the parasitic factor, we must consider the predisposing factors that cause the skin (suitable soil) to be suitable for parasitic infestation or harmful effects. Without such a causative factor, even if a parasitic agent is present on the skin, it will not be pathogenic (disease development).

The most common causes are constipation and digestive disorders, which are easily recognized by the patients themselves. Indulgence in indigestible food, beer, or other alcoholic beverages at night or during the day often kills new eruptions in those with this tendency.

Not only do I not wish to bore the reader with further lengthy quotations from the famous dermatological treatises, but also because many readers believe that the specialty is often narrowly prejudiced, I will only add two medical doctors, Dr. Combs and Dr. Bryce, to my sister. These two represent the opinions of prominent surgeons. One of the most detestable skin diseases is anal pruritus, i.e., prurigo of the anus. This pruritus is so severe that the patient cannot sleep, is lulled into despair, and sometimes goes into insanity. When internal medicine and dermatology are unable to help, the patient is referred to surgery. The surgeon will remove a large piece of skin as a last resort to stop the intolerable pruritus. Pruritus, like most dermatoses and other diseases of the body, is the result of a combination of improper nutrition and stagnant elimination. It is not a single localized dermatosis, as it begins with stomach and intestinal problems and spreads to other parts of the body, manifesting itself as a multitude of symptoms. Pruritic patients are usually victims of gout, leumatism, cystitis, diabetes mellitus, liver disease, etc., and the new disease is the result of malnutrition and defecation, as will be shown elsewhere. The renowned surgeon J. B. Lockhart-Mummery, in his famous book "Diseases of the Rectum and Colon," pp. 602 and 605 (J. P. Lockhart-Mummery: - Diseases of the Rectum and Colon, p. 602, 605.)

Proctoptosis is a unique disease that develops only one symptom: pruritus. It has no properly proven pathology. We are still groping in the dark as to its cause or the best way to replace it. This is by no means a minor disorder, as the name implies. In some cases, the pruritus may become so intense and almost glowing that the patient is driven to the brink of madness.

The rash is far more common in boys than in girls. However, this is not to say that it is rare among girls. According to Dr. Adler of Philadelphia, ninety-five percent of the patients he has treated in his practice for pruritus were boys. In my own experience, however, I cannot say that boys account for such a large proportion.

Prurigo is extremely common in hypervirulent people who habitually overeat and overeat. If such patients follow a strict regimen, their condition is always improved. In simpler terms, there is no doubt that prurigo and indigestion are inextricably linked.

There are some patients who suffer from prurigo as a result of overeating certain foods. Some say that they always get prurigo when they eat shellfish. Other patients say they get itching when they drink too much alcohol, tea, or coffee, and in some patients, excessive smoking can cause the same result.

As mentioned above, both skin specialists and non-specialists generally attribute the cause of skin diseases to digestive disorders. However, they do not seem to understand the root cause. However, it has been their practical experience that when they are forced to use conventional laxatives, it becomes a habit, and they later find that there is nothing they can do about it. In the case of the conventional laxative, the patient is suddenly faced with a "dilemma. The laxative itself is good, but the addictive nature of the laxative eventually leads to the worst, and the conclusion is that there is no other way but to have the patient cured by surgery. This is a mistake. The actual purpose of Tetrapathy is not only to directly eliminate intestinal fecal retention, but also to remove the remote cause of the retention, and at the same time to restore, correct, repair, reinforce, and heal the paralysis, swelling, hemorrhage, and laceration of the cerebral vessels caused by feces and its accompanying auto-poisoning. This is what we should call the true fundamental therapy. The drug Klimag (Milk of Magnesia) was devised to work in the same way as this natural method, and to eliminate defecation without any side effects. Dr. Höller's efforts were truly worthwhile, and my own path was the same. Therefore, I personally supervised, enjoyed, and released a drug that can be safely taken and removed by any person.

Concluding Words

To have beautiful skin, you must have enough bowel movements at least twice a day. For those who are suffering from skin diseases, the first step is to use Climagogue (Milk of Magnesia brand) to control the circulation. The dosage can be freely determined, so at first, dissolve a few teaspoons in a glass of clear water, stir well, and drink on an empty stomach. If there is no effect, increase the dose; if there is too much, decrease the dose. If the same dosage is not effective, the dosage should be increased; if it is too much, the dosage should be decreased. After a while, as early as a week, the stools may be black or brown in color, mixed with bugs, lumpy with bugs, singing, watery, or in a variety of other states, but there is no need to worry about weakness. In such cases, they should chew their normal diet more carefully than usual. In this case, the patient should be given a few months of fretfulness, as an example.

When taking a bath, mix a few spoonful of kurimag in a bathtub of cold or hot water and bathe hot or cold, and practice the following

six major rules, agar, wind therapy, etc.

Six Major Laws of Health

First, Sleeping on hard floor

Second, Sleeping on hard pillow therapy

Third, goldfish exercise

Fourth, capillary exercise therapy

Fifth, Hand cure

Sixth, the dorso-ventral exercise

For more information on the above six laws,

agar diet, air bath therapy, etc., please refer to

page 211 and following of my book, "Secrets

of Fighting Disease".